Manage Cholesterol naturally

And

Prevent Heart attacks

By

V.K.Grover

DISCLAIMER AND/OR LEGAL NOTICES

The information within this book is intended as reference materials only and not as medical or professional advice. Information contained herein is intended to give you the tools to make informed decisions about your lifestyle and health. It should not be used as a substitute for any treatment that has been prescribed or recommended by your doctor. The information presented herein represents the views of the author. This book is the outcome of my study of **alternative medicines** including Natural treatments for more than 20 years.

Why you need this book

This book is the outcome of my study of **alternative medicines** including Natural treatments for more than 20 years.

About 40% of people have high cholesterol, but many of them are unaware of the same. It is said that high cholesterol can lead to heart problem. Purpose of the book is to inform about the correct position of same. The book deals with methods of controlling the LDL naturally, increasing HDL and avoid the side effects of medicines.

Heart Disease is the second cause of death in America.

The ideas in this book will help you lower your cholesterol and prevent Heart Attacks. Use and apply all the tips and advice that you find useful for controlling your Cholesterol and prevent Heart Attacks.

Several things may contribute to high cholesterol, and several things can help lower it. The steps that must be taken vary with each person. This book simply gives you the tools you need to develop your own program for a healthy cholesterol level.

Please be advised that the advice and tips contained here are for help to manage your Cholesterol but consult a doctor before following these recommendations.

The information within this book is intended as reference materials only and not as medical or professional advice. Information contained herein is intended to give you the tools to make informed decisions about your lifestyle and health. It should not be used as a substitute for any treatment that has been prescribed or recommended by your doctor. The information presented herein represents the views of the author.

I hope that this book will help the readers to remain healthy and disease free. I shall be very happy if suggestions and methods given can help you in management of Cholesterol and prevention of Heart Attack.

Thanks

I am grateful to God who inspired me to write this book.

I am also thankful to my wife and children and friends for their love and support, without which it would not have been possible to write this book.

Contents

Chapter 1

Introduction

Cholesterol is a soft, wax like substance that exists throughout the body. It is an important part of the body that is required for the maintenance of the body. But it is also supposed to be the greatest silent killer. Most of the doctors believe that high levels of cholesterol can cause heart attacks but some others believe that the attacks are not due to cholesterol but due to inflammation of arteries. But it is accepted even by these researchers that Cholesterol can cause inflammation. So directly or indirectly cholesterol is an important factor for heart attacks.

Cholesterol is created in the liver, almost three grams daily, and then sent into the blood stream. Here it mixes with proteins to form lipoproteins which make it water soluble and usable by the cells. Cholesterol then forms a waterproof barrier around cells to protect them from viruses and other harmful organisms. It is essential in the production of many hormones, most importantly the creation of the male hormone, testosterone. It surrounds and protects each and every cell in the body, including a large portion of the brain, playing a significant role in the construction of synapses, the body structure through which messages are sent from the brain to other parts of the body. Cholesterol is essential for body functions including formation of cells, protection of nerve tissue, brain cells, digestion and manufacturing of hormones. We cannot live without it. It is practically in every part of our body. Not only is cholesterol needed in all of these instances, but also it is a building block for the growth of foetal cells and production of vitamin D. It is   an important ingredient in digestive juices.

It is important that levels of Cholesterol are maintained in proper level as less amount can create problem of growth but too much cholesterol in the body can cause damage by clogging arteries. This puts you at serious risk for disease such as heart and stroke. In fact, the major cause behind heart attacks and strokes is clogged arteries resulting from high levels of cholesterol. Cholesterol is also associated with memory disorders such as dementia and Alzheimer's disease.

Diet plays an important part in the levels of Cholesterol. When you eat saturated foods such as dairy, meat and eggs your cholesterol level goes up. On the other hand when you eat foods such as fruits, vegetables, and grains you can maintain optimal health as they do not contain cholesterol. With proper nutritious diet high cholesterol can be avoided. This book deals with most of these extraordinary methods of treatment and can help readers in their pursuit for healthy life.

Chapter2

Types of Cholesterol

Just like all fats, cholesterol doesn't dissolve in the blood. Therefore, if it wants to travel around the body to get where it needs to go, it has to be carried. To get to and from your cells, cholesterol is transported by "carriers" called lipoproteins.

The "density" of lipoproteins is measured by the amount of protein in the molecule. There are mainly two types of Cholesterol namely LDL and HDL. There is one more type of Cholesterol namely VLDL.VLDL is called Triglycerides. However VLDL, LDL and HDL are not actually cholesterol. They are the lipoproteins that carry cholesterol through the blood. LDL is a low density lipoprotein that carries cholesterol from the liver to tissues while HDL is a high density lipoprotein that carries cholesterol away from tissues and back to the liver to be metabolized and reused.

LDL has less protein but is high in cholesterol while HDL has lower amounts of cholesterol but is high in protein. With this, LDL causes clogging of the artery and the HDL is the one responsible in clearing the bad form of cholesterol that comes from the bloodstream.

• Very-low-density lipoprotein (VLDL). This type of lipoprotein contains the most triglycerides, a type of fat, attached to the proteins in your blood. VLDL cholesterol makes LDL cholesterol larger in size, causing your blood vessels to narrow. If you're taking cholesterol-lowering medication but have a high VLDL level, you may need additional medication to lower your triglycerides.

Triglycerides are necessary for good health. Your body uses them for energy. But high triglycerides can also raise your risk of heart disease and may be a sign of metabolic syndrome that is the combination of high blood pressure, high blood sugar, and too much fat around the waist, low HDL and high triglycerides. Metabolic syndrome increases your risk for stroke.

HDL is considered the "good" cholesterol because it actually helps protect your body by transporting cholesterol away from your arteries. HDL [high density lipoprotein) is considered to be the good one as its particles prevent atherosclerosis by extracting cholesterol from the artery walls and then disposing of them through the liver. There are several methods for increasing the good cholesterol.

LDL is considered the "bad" cholesterol because it is largely responsible for the negative effects cholesterol has on your health. High levels of LDL tend to clog up the inner walls of important arteries, including those that send blood to the brain and heart. LDL cholesterol is responsible for the buildup of plaque that can lead to heart attacks and stroke.

Cholesterol is typically measured in three different ways:

Total cholesterol,

LDL cholesterol and

HDL cholesterol.

LDL/HDL ratio

LDL/ Total cholesterol ratio.

Cholesterol levels will fall within one of three categories
Desirable, Borderline and High Risk.

Following gives the values for these risks.

Cholesterol Type	Desirable	Borderline	High Risk
Total Cholesterol	Below 200	200-240	Above 240
HDL Cholesterol	Above 45	35-45	Below 35
LDL Cholesterol	Below 130	130-160	Above 160
Total/ HDL	Below 4.5	4.5-5.5	Above 5.5
LDL/HDL	Below 3	3-5	Above 5

Triglycerides	Below 150	150-199	Above 200

Less than one half of adults in America have a cholesterol level of 200 and below. If your total cholesterol numbers read less than 200,
chances are good that your risk of a heart attack is relatively low (This risk level could be increased if you have other risk factors). However, even if your numbers suggest a low risk, you should still begin thinking about the food choices you make and assess your level of exercise. A lifestyle of low cholesterol foods and a high level of physical activity will help assure you of a healthier and happier life.

Borderline

If your total cholesterol levels are between 200to 239, you are considered borderline or borderline-high risk. If you are in this group, you are not necessarily at high risk for heart disease. However, if you fall in this group, it is recommended to follow a diet and exercise plan to control the levels especially if you are at risk because of other factors like hereditary. Your goal should be to bring these values in safer range.

High Risk

If your total cholesterol level is 240 or higher, you are definitely at risk of stroke, heart attack, and other complications of heart disease. Researchers estimate that people who have a total cholesterol level in this range are more than two times more likely to suffer a heart attack than people with a cholesterol level in the desirable range. Your doctor will most likely have a plan of action to help you lower your cholesterol, including diet, exercise, and possibly medication.

CHAPTER 3

Factors of High Cholesterol

Factors within your control such as inactivity, obesity and an unhealthy diet — contribute to high LDL cholesterol and low HDL cholesterol. Factors beyond your control may play a role, too. For example, your genetic makeup may keep cells from removing LDL cholesterol from your blood efficiently or cause your liver to produce too much cholesterol

There are numerous factors that play a role in cholesterol level. These factors are age, diet, disease, gender, genetics, lifestyle, and weight

Age

The average human's blood cholesterol levels increase with age.

With increased blood cholesterol levels, the categories of Desirable, Borderline, and High Risk become less important. Your primary care physician will likely take your age into consideration when assessing your cholesterol levels and developing a plan o f action for your situation.

Diet

Your diet is one of the most important factors leading to your cholesterol level. A diet that contains foods high in saturated fats trans-fats and that is high in cholesterol can lead to Hypercholesterolemia and may result in severe damage, including atherosclerosis, coronary heart disease, and stroke. Eating foods that contain high levels of cholesterol, especially when combined with foods high in saturated fats and trans-fats can lead to potentially dangerous cholesterol rates.

Diseases

A number of diseases can heighten your risk of high cholesterol. Diseases such as Diabetes and hypertension play a key role in speeding up the atherosclerosis. Increased pressure on your artery walls because of high blood pressure damages your arteries, which can speed the accumulation of fatty deposits.

High blood sugar contributes to higher LDL cholesterol and lower HDL cholesterol. High blood sugar also damages the lining of your arteries.

Ironically, some of the medications (notably beta-blockers) that are used to treat hypertension can actually increase your levels of LDL and triglycerides as they decrease your HDL.

Gender

As a fact of nature, men seem to have higher LDL levels and lower HDL levels than women. This is especially true in both men and women under the age of 5o. However, post-menopausal women tend to have increased levels of LDL— this as per researchers is due to decreased levels of estrogen being produced by a woman's body during this period of her life.

Genetics

It is not completely understood but it is observed that genetic defects passed between parents and children can lead to either a higher production of LDL or a lessened ability for the body to remove the LDL. That means when your parents have displayed signs of high cholesterol, it is best to get yourself checked to assess your current level of risk.

If a parent or sibling developed heart disease before age 55, high cholesterol levels place you at a greater than average risk of developing heart disease.

Lifestyle

High stress, inactivity, and smoking can all raise your total cholesterol level.

Exercise:

Helps you in your goal of control of cholesterol. Exercise does not need to be an enormous undertaking; workouts of less than an hour each day can make a significant difference. One study showed that when the more than 700 subjects exercised for 40 minutes a day, their HDL gains were significant enough to translate to a 5 to 7% drop in overall heart disease risk. In this same study, conducted at the University of Tokyo, the minimum time spent exercising each week that was required to change HDL levels was 120 minutes You only have to carve out workout for 40 minutes a day for three days each week to see a change. In fact, researchers found that working out for a full 40 minutes was more important than how often or how hard the participants worked out.

While daily outs are best, there is no harm in taking a couple of work days off. Just be sure to get at least 30 to 40 minutes of exercise during each workout, or extend them to an hour or more to get even better results.You do not have to break records for speed or strength when choosing your activity. Exercise should be a part of your regular routine. It is better to choose an activity that you enjoy so that you can stick with. Dancing, brisk walking, bicycling and even vigorous gardening -- anything that gets the heart rate up-- can all be great ways to enjoy the time you spend exercising. If you get bored with an activity, just switch to something else. What is important is that you get moving and keep moving. Remember, the intensity of the workout does not matter as much as the duration of the exercise you are doing. In other words, your 30+ minutes a day are beneficial whether you spend them jumping over hurdles or walking -- so do something you will enjoy on a regular basis.

Weight

Overweight people are much more likely to have high levels of cholesterol than people at healthy body weights. In addition, overweight and obese individuals typically have lower HDL levels.

It is, of course, important to remember that these factors all exist together. In other words, if you are an overweight, smoker with hypertension and a history of high cholesterol in your family, your risk of heart attack could dramatically increase. On the other hand, if you are an athletic individual who eats well, but have family history of high cholesterol, your diet and exercise might just keep you safe. If you want to take control of your cholesterol levels you should care all areas of your life.

Cholesterol risk factors can be avoided through healthy life style and taking proper diet.

Chapter 4

Risk of Heart attack

What Is Your Risk of Developing Heart Disease or Having a Heart Attack?

In general, the higher your LDL level and the more risk factors you have (other than LDL), the greater your chances of developing heart disease or having a heart attack. Some people are at high risk for a heart attack because they already have heart disease. Other people are at high risk for developing heart disease because they have diabetes (which is a strong risk factor) or a combination of risk factors for heart disease. Follow these steps to find out your risk for developing heart disease.

Step 1: Check the table below to see how many of the listed risk factors you have; these are the risk factors that affect your LDL goal.

Major Risk Factors That Affect Your LDL Goal

•   Cigarette smoking
•   High blood pressure (140/90 mmHg or higher or on blood pressure medication)
•   Low HDL cholesterol (less than 40 mg/dL)*
•   Family history of early heart disease (heart disease in father or brother before age 55; heart disease in mother or sister before age 65)
•   Age (men 45 years or older; women 55 years or older)

* If your HDL cholesterol is 60 mg/dl or higher, subtract 1 from your total count.

Even though obesity and physical inactivity are not counted in this list, they are conditions that need to be corrected.

Step 2: How many major risk factors do you have? If you have 2 or more risk factors in the table above, use the attached risk scoring tables (which include your cholesterol levels) to find your risk score. Risk score refers to the chance of having a heart attack in the next 10 years, given as a percentage. My risk score is _____%.

Step 3: Use your medical history, number of risk factors, and risk score to find your risk of developing heart disease or having a heart attack in the table below.

If You Have	You Are in Category
Heart disease, diabetes, or risk score more than 20%*	I. High Risk
2 or more risk factors and risk score 10-20%	II. Next Highest Risk
2 or more risk factors and risk score less than 10%	III. Moderate Risk
0 or 1 risk factor	IV. Low-to-Moderate Risk

* Means that more than 20 of 100 people in this category will have a heart attack within 10 years.

My risk category is _____.

Estimate of 10-Year Risk for Men

Framingham Point Scores by Age Group

Age	Points
20-34	-9
35-39	-4
40-44	0
45-49	3
50-54	6
55-59	8
60-64	10
65-69	11

70-74	12
75-79	13

Framingham Point Scores by Age Group and Total Cholesterol

Total Cholesterol	Age 20-39	Age 40-49	Age 50-59	Age 60-69	Age 70-79
<160	0	0	0	0	0
160-199	4	3	2	1	0
200-239	7	5	3	1	0
240-279	9	6	4	2	1
280+	11	8	5	3	1

Framingham Point Scores by Age and Smoking Status

	Age 20	Age 40	Age 50	Age 60	Age 70

	-39	-49	-59	-69	-79
Nonsmoker	0	0	0	0	0
Smoker	8	5	3	1	1

Framingham Point Scores by HDL Level

HDL	Points
60+	-1
50-59	0
40-49	1
<40	2

Framingham Point Scores by Systolic Blood Pressure and Treatment Status

Systolic BP	If Untreated	If Treated
<120	0	0

120-129	0	1
130-139	1	2
140-159	1	2
160+	2	3

10-Year Risk by Total Framingham Point Scores

Point Total	10-Year Risk
< 0	< 1%
0	1%
1	1%
2	1%
3	1%
4	1%

5	2%
6	2%
7	3%
8	4%
9	5%
10	6%
11	8%
12	10%
13	12%
14	16%
15	20%
16	25%
17 or more	$\geq 30\%$

Estimate of 10-Year Risk for Women

Framingham Point Scores by Age Group

Age	Points
20-34	-7
35-39	-3
40-44	0
45-49	3
50-54	6
55-59	8
60-64	10
65-69	12
70-74	14
75-79	16

Framingham Point Scores by Age Group and Total Cholesterol

Total Cholesterol	Age 20-39	Age 40-49	Age 50-59	Age 60-69	Age 70-79
<160	0	0	0	0	0
160-199	4	3	2	1	1
200-239	8	6	4	2	1
240-279	11	8	5	3	2
280+	13	10	7	4	2

Framingham Point Scores by Age and Smoking Status

	Age 20-39	Age 40-49	Age 50-59	Age 60-69	Age 70-79
Nonsmoker	0	0	0	0	0

Smoker	9	7	4	2	1	

Framingham Point Scores by HDL Level

HDL	Points
60+	-1
50-59	0
40-49	1
<40	2

Framingham Point Scores by Systolic Blood Pressure and Treatment Status

Systolic BP	If Untreated	If Treated
<120	0	0
120-	1	3

129		
130-139	2	4
140-159	3	5
160+	4	6

10-Year Risk by Total Framingham Point Scores

Point Total	10-Year Risk
< 9	< 1%
9	1%
10	1%
11	1%
12	1%
13	2%
14	2%

15	3%
16	4%
17	5%
18	6%
19	8%
20	11%
21	14%
22	17%
23	22%
24	27%
25 or more	≥30%

If you are in

•   **Category I, Highest Risk**, your LDL goal is less than 100 mg/dl you will need to begin the

TLC diet to reduce your high risk even if your LDL is below 100 mg/dl. If your LDL is 100 or above, you will need to start drug treatment at the same time as the TLC diet. If your LDL is below 100 mg/dl, you may also need to start drug treatment together with the TLC diet if your doctor finds your risk is very high, for example if you had a recent heart attack or have both heart disease and diabetes.

• **Category II, Next Highest Risk**, your LDL goal is less than 130 mg/dl.

• If your LDL is 130 mg/dl or above, you will need to begin treatment with the TLC diet. If your LDL is 130 mg/dl or more after 3 months on the TLC diet, you may need drug treatment along with the TLC diet. If your LDL is less than 130 mg/dl, you will need to follow the heart healthy diet which allows a little more saturated fat and cholesterol than the TLC diet.

• **Category III, Moderate Risk**, your LDL goal is less than 130 mg/dl.

• If your LDL is 130 mg/dl or above, you will need to begin the TLC diet. If your LDL is 160 mg/dl or more after you have tried the TLC diet for 3 months, you may need drug treatment along with the TLC diet. If your LDL is less than 130 mg/dl, you will need to follow the heart healthy diet.

• **Category IV, Low-to-Moderate Risk**, your LDL goal is less than 160 mg/dl.

• If your LDL is 160 mg/dl or above, you will need to begin the TLC diet. If your LDL is still 160 mg/dl or more after 3 months on the TLC diet, you may need drug treatment along with the TLC diet to lower your LDL, especially if your LDL is 190 mg/dl or more. If your LDL is less than 160 mg/dl, you will need to follow the heart healthy diet.

To reduce your risk for heart disease or keep it low, it is very important to control any other risk factors you may have such as high blood pressure and smoking.

Lowering Cholesterol with Therapeutic Lifestyle Changes (TLC)

TLC is a set of things you can do to help lower your LDL cholesterol. The main parts of TLC are:

• *The TLC Diet.* This is a low-saturated-fat, low-cholesterol eating plan that calls for less than 7percent of calories from saturated fat and less than 200 mg of dietary cholesterol per day. The TLC diet recommends only enough calories to maintain a desirable weight and avoid weight gain. If your LDL is not lowered enough by reducing your saturated fat and cholesterol intakes, the amount of soluble fiber in your diet can be increased. Certain food products that contain plant stanols or plant sterols (for example, cholesterol-lowering margarines) can also be added to the TLC diet to boost its LDL-lowering power.

• *Weight Management.* Losing weight if you are overweight can help lower LDL and is especially important for those with a cluster of risk factors that includes high triglyceride and/or low HDL levels and being overweight with a large waist measurement (more than 40 inches for men and more than 35 inches for women).

• *Physical Activity.* Regular physical activity (30 minutes on most, if not all, days) is recommended for everyone. It can help raise HDL and lower LDL and is especially important for those with high triglyceride and/or low HDL levels who are overweight with a large waist measurement.

Drug Treatment

Even if you begin drug treatment to lower your cholesterol, you will need to continue your treatment with lifestyle changes. This will keep the dose of medicine as low as possible, and lower your risk in other ways as well. There are several types of drugs available for cholesterol lowering including statins, bile acid sequestrants, nicotinic acid, fibric acids, and cholesterol absorption inhibitors. Your doctor can help decide which type of drug is best for you. The statin drugs are very effective in lowering LDL levels and are safe for most people. Bile acid sequestrants also lower LDL and can be used alone or in combination with statin drugs. Nicotinic acid lowers LDL and triglycerides and raises HDL. Fibric acids lower LDL somewhat but are used mainly to treat high triglyceride and low HDL levels. Cholesterol absorption inhibitors lower LDL and can be used alone or in combination with statin drugs.

Once your LDL goal has been reached, your doctor may prescribe treatment for high triglycerides and/or a low HDL level, if present. The treatment includes losing weight if needed, increasing physical activity, quitting smoking, and possibly taking a drug.

Chapter 5

Treating High Cholesterol through life change

The main goal of cholesterol-lowering treatment is to lower your LDL and Triglycides levels enough to reduce your risk of developing heart disease or having a heart attack. The higher your risk, the lower your LDL goal will be. To find your LDL goal, see the boxes below for your risk category. There are two main ways to lower your cholesterol:

• Therapeutic Lifestyle Changes (TLC)-- includes a cholesterol-lowering diet (called the TLC diet), physical activity, and weight management. TLC is for anyone whose LDL is above goal.

•   Drug Treatment--if cholesterol-lowering drugs are needed, they are used together with TLC treatment to help lower your LDL.

Prevention

You Are What You Eat

Luckily, reducing your cholesterol can sometimes be as easy as changing what you eat. Since most instances of high cholesterol are a result of your dietary cholesterol (the stuff you eat) rather than your blood cholesterol (the cholesterol your body produces), a change in diet can often have a profound effect on your cholesterol levels.

The most expedient way to reduce your cholesterol levels is by cutting out, or reducing, the foods you eat that contain high levels of saturated fat and/or cholesterol. However, you'll need to be more specific than this in your diet to begin lowering your cholesterol. To lower your cholesterol, you will need to know both the foods you should avoid and the foods you should eat. Of course, to create the best plan for your needs, you should consult your primary care physician/dietician before starting any new diet plan.

Foods to AVOID if You Want to Lower Your Cholesterol

If you are serious about lowering your cholesterol, there is a list of foods and food types that you should avoid at all costs. Foods to avoid:

1. Any foods that contain high amounts of saturated fat, such as marbled, poultry with skin, and full-fat dairy products

As you now know, saturated fat plays a main role in increasing your cholesterol levels. Researchers have proven that lowering your intake of saturated fats will lower LDL (bad) cholesterol levels.

2. Any foods that contain high levels of cholesterol, such as dairy products (e.g., eggs, cheese and sour cream), meats with high saturated fat, and poultry

Health experts advise that your daily diet should contain no more than 300 milligrams of cholesterol. This number, of course, will vary based on the specific individual. You should always consult your primary care physician to determine the appropriate level for yourself.

3. Any foods that contain high levels of trans -fat, such as cakes, cookies, crackers, and fried foods

Health experts advise that your daily diet should contain no more than 1% trans- fat.

4. Any meats that contain high levels of fat, such as corned beef, pastrami, ribs, steak, ground meat, frankfurters, sausage, bacon, liver, kidneys, and processed meats like bologna.

Foods that are prepared in any of the following ways are often high in fat:

Fried, basted, braised, au gratin, crispy, escalloped, pan-fried, sautéed stewed or stuffed foods. These are generally all high sources of fat.

5. Any foods that are high in sodium, such foods that are pickled, smoked, or salted

While discussion is still ongoing as to the effects of sodium as it relates to hypertension, there is no harm in being proactive and moderating your sodium just to be safe. Remember, hypertension can speed up the progression of atherosclerosis.

6. As far as possible, avoid fast foods, including hamburgers, fries, fried chicken, and tacos.

Most fast foods are high in total fat, saturated fats, trans- fats, and hydrogenated fats. And, remember, the cheese and mayonnaise-based dressings of many fast food products make their fat and cholesterol levels that much higher.

> 7. Foods that are high in refined sugars and carbohydrates

Sugars tend to limit the ability of your body to effectively process a number of cholesterol fighting helpers, such as vitamin C and Rice Bran Extract IP6. A low carbohydrate diet high in fiber and low in sugar and fats, especially trans- fats, is superb way to increase your dietary fiber intake while avoiding the negatives of refined sugars.

Foods You Can Eat to Lower Your Cholesterol

Just as there are certain foods that you should definitely avoid, there are others that you should make a part of your daily diet. These foods include:

8. Fiber-rich foods, including fruits, vegetables, beans, and oats Fiber-rich foods have actually been shown to help lower your cholesterol. In addition, because fiber gives you the sensation of being full, it is also been found to help in weight control. Health experts suggest your daily diet contain 25 to 38 grams of fiber.
9. Fish, including flounder, trout, tuna, halibut, and salmon

Many types of fish are low in saturated fat and high in healthy omega-3 fatty acids. Health experts suggest a diet that contains no less than two servings of grilled or baked fish a week.

10. Soy foods, including soy milk and soy burgers

Health experts suggest a daily diet that includes 25 grams of soy protein each day.

11. Foods that contain monounsaturated fats, such as avocados and olive oil

When eating out, be sure to look for dishes that have been baked, broiled, grilled, poached, roasted, or steamed. These dishes will likely be lower in total cholesterol because they were not cooked in fatty oils. Be sure to ask your server for details.

12. If you choose to eat meat, choose lower fat options, such as skinless chicken, lean beef, veal, pork, and lamb. But as far as possible try to avoid these foods.

Most important factor for lowering Cholesterol is change in diet.

HEART UK, has identified "six super foods" that actively lower cholesterol levels:

- Soya foods (15g a day) - soya milk, soya desserts, soya meat alternatives, soya nuts, edamame beans and tofu
- Nuts - a handful a day
- Oats and barley - providing the soluble fiber beta glucan
- Plant sterols/stanols - found in a wide range of foods
- Fruits and vegetables
- Foods rich in unsaturated fats - for example, canola and vegetable oils.

HEART UK also lists foods that are bad for cholesterol levels:

.

- Ghee
- Hard margarines
- Lard
- Fatty and processed meat
- Dairy fats.

CHAPTER 6

Treating High Cholesterol through other natural means

In this chapter we will discuss some natural ways to lower cholesterol and keep it down. While proper diet and exercise is critical to your overall health and reducing your cholesterol levels, these natural actions will help your body to establish the proper levels of cholesterol. We encourage you to discuss these practices with your physician before implementing into your daily regime.

Diet:

Besides the above Foods the following natural treatments should be used to control Cholesterol

1. Drink Milk' Unhomogenized/skimmed

Milk being an animal product contains fats and cholesterol and is not the healthy choice for a person with high cholesterol.

Researchers are beginning to evaluate claims that milk in itself might not present the cholesterol-raising properties it was once thought to have. Evidence suggests that the process of homogenization actually may be milk's main offender.

Milk has two components. If you put the container having milk in a refrigerator, you'd end up with two layers— skim milk would be at the bottom of the container and a layer of cream would sit at the top. By its definition, skim milk has no fat while cream is basically all fat. Without homogenization, all milk would either be skim or cream or a mixture of both that would always separate when it settles. The process of homogenization takes the cream and breaks it down, so that it can stay mixed with the milk. This is how we have whole milk and milks with a variety of fat precents (e.g., 1%, 2%).

As homogenization process is breaking down the fat (cream) into much smaller molecules, it is actually increasing the milk fat's surface area. With the surface area of the fats increased, it can do more damage to the arterial walls. Increased damage, such as plaque build-up and scraping of existing plaque, can lead to a clogging of the arteries and/or a break-free of plaque that could cause strokes.

It means that when your cholesterol levels are high, choosing fat of any kind is not recommended. It is advised to drink fat-free and/or unhomogenized milk/skimmed milk.

Note: If you buy unhomogenized milk, be sure to remove the cream layer as this is very high in fat. Better if you buy skimmed milk only.

2. Supplement with Vitamin C

It seems that vitamin C, an antioxidant, is good for just about all that ails, including cholesterol, too. Research is showing that vitamin C, taken regularly, can actually help in reduction of cholesterol.

When levels of vitamin C are low, your body compensates by manufacturing more cholesterol. However, when vitamin C levels are high, the vitamin helps to lower cholesterol.

According to a recent study published in the American Journal of Clinical Nutrition, studies have shown that individuals who take more than 700 mg of vitamin C daily can reduce their risk of heart disease over those who don't. For lowering cholesterol, individual dosages will vary depending on the cholesterol level. Although the Recommended Daily Allowance is only under 100mg for most people, according to the American Academy of Family Physicians (AAFP), a dosage of 500 mg of vitamin C twice a day is considered "reasonable." In addition, there are those in the medical field who suggest much higher daily doses of 1000mg and more. It is best to consult with your physician to establish the ideal recommended daily dosage for you.

Recent studies confirm the theories of Nobel prize-winning scientist Linus Pauling that vitamin C taken in concert with lysine and proline have a potentially profound impact on lowering cholesterol by helping to remove plaque from your arteries. More specifically, Pauling's The Natural Cure for Heart Disease states that 6g to 18g of Vitamin C taken as Ascorbic Acid with/or before meals (e.g., 2 to 3 times daily) with 3g to 6g Lysine, .5g-2g Proline, and 150 mg-3oo mg CoQio can have an intensely positive effect on cholesterol and plaque levels.

Pauling claims that by using a high vitamin C and lysine therapy "Heart Disease can be successfully treated, without surgery or prescription" His quick and easy treatments put the power of healing right in your hands

3. Limit Your Intake of Sugar and Refined Carbohydrates as it is proven that Sugar could be keeping your cholesterol levels higher than they need to be.

As you just read, vitamin C can have a positive effect on lowering your risk of heart disease and actively lowering your cholesterol, sugar and refined carbohydrates, particularly glucose, limits the beneficial effects that vitamin C provides

Because we typically have such high levels of glucose in our bodies, it affects the absorption of Vitamin C and prevents healing and protection from the dangerous effects of cholesterol. These refined sugars actually slow down the response and effectiveness of your immune system, not only to the effects of cholesterol damage, but also to everything from the common cold to much more severe viruses.

Rice Bran Extract IP6 is known to significantly reduce cholesterol, but the amount of sugar you consume inhibits the beneficial properties of cholesterol-fighting IP6. Cutting back on refined sugars will increase your body's ability to best use IP6 and help you begin lowering your cholesterol immediately.

So, the next time you're considering eating highly refined sugars in the forms of sucrose (table sugar), dextrose (corn sugar), and high-fructose corn, think of the fact that you are robbing your body's immune system of the true fuel it needs, like vitamin C.

4. Fiber diet

Numerous studies have shown that eating high fiber foods, such as apples, will reduce LDL cholesterol. Other high fiber foods that are particularly beneficial include oat products and legumes (dry beans, peas, and lentils). Drinking fibre solutions that contain psyllium have also been found advantageous.

A low carbohydrate diet high in fibre and low in sugar and fats is a superb way to increase your dietary fibre intake while avoiding the negatives of refined sugars. Low carb diet that includes ample servings of fruits and vegetables on a daily basis is an excellent way to improve overall health and help reduce the negative effects of LDL cholesterol.

5.   Taurine

Research and numerous studies have shown that taurine, an amino acid can have an especially beneficial effect on cholesterol levels. Taurine works by increasing gallbladder function and reducing LDL and increasing HDL cholesterol. In fact, taurine taking 1500 to 3000 milligrams daily has been shown to raise good cholesterol level by as much as 25% by. Dosage will depend on situation.

Besides lowering cholesterol taurine plays a role in memory, aging, eye, heart, and skin health, as well as hypertension and Cystic Fibrosis.

7.   Rice Bran Extract IP6

IP6 is a Phytic acid and is found in every cell of the human body. It is also found in whole grains, seeds, and nuts. IP6 is a mineral chelator and it acts as a cleansing agent in the body, removing harmful build-up of heavy metals and other accumulations, including those found in our arteries. IP6 derived from rice bran has been documented to reduce and inhibit calcifications throughout the body, including within the arteries. According to the International Journal Cardiology, IP6 can "potentially remove calcium deposits from arteries." Research shows the positive effects IP6 can have on individuals with high cholesterol.

While the proper dosages will vary from person to person, taking 2000 mg of oral IP6 rice bran extract on an empty stomach with water once a day for 30 days once a year seems to have shown beneficial results. In addition, because of its chelating effects, this procedure is thought to clean out the liver of excess iron as well.

Note: Pregnant women, children who have high iron needs, and anaemic individuals should avoid using this product. As with any new health regimen, consult your primary care physician before beginning.

8.   Rice Bran Oil

Recent research shows that rice bran oil actually reduces LDL cholesterol without reducing HDL cholesterol. Interestingly, rice bran oil contains the antioxidants tocopherol, oryzanol, and tocotrienol from the vitamin E family.

Given the amazing cholesterol-lowering properties of rice bran oil, switching from other vegetable oils like corn, soy, safflower, and canola is highly recommended.

9. Change Your Diet

Eliminate saturated fats and trans-fats from your diet. Foods that have saturated fats are marbled meats, poultry with skin on, and full fat dairy products.

Trans fats are directly associated with heart disease and with increasing the LDL cholesterol that leads to clogged arteries. While totally eliminating trans-fats from your diet might be very difficult, experts agree that a diet that consists of no more than 1% trans-fat within your total daily allowance should suffice. You should go out of your way to determine which foods contain trans-fats and avoid them.

Trans-fats are normally found in foods made with or cooked in hydrogenated vegetable oil. Examples of these foods include crackers and fried snack foods, such as potato chips. Baked goods, such as cookies, cakes, and doughnuts also contain trans-fats. Even foods labelled "low in cholesterol" or "low in saturated fats" could still contain trans-fats. In addition, many margarines and hydrogenated vegetable shortening contains trans- fats. Trans-fats are also found naturally in some meats and dairy products.

The easiest way to determine if a packaged food has trans-fats or not is to read the label and, if you see the words "hydrogenated" or "partially hydrogenated" it means that it contains trans-fats.

10. Pomegranate

Studies have shown that the incredible antioxidant properties of pomegranate juice can help lower cholesterol. Pomegranate juice has been found to reduce the oxidation of LDL and lowering the risk of atherosclerosis. Pomegranate juice is very good source of phytochemical compounds. (Substances that are beneficial to the heart and blood vessels.) Recently concluded studies gave heart patients an ounce of pomegranate juice every day for a year. The blood pressure of the participants lowered by over 20% and there was 30% reduction in atherosclerotic plaque. It is advised to drink pomegranate juice every day.

11. Vitamin E

Vitamin E is very good for reducing LDL. The vitamin E family contains tocopherols and tocotrienols and each of these has four forms: alpha, beta, gamma, and delta.

Delta tocotrienol is noted for having the strongest cholesterol-lowering properties.

In a study by the Kenneth Jordan Heart Foundation, palm-based tocotrienols showed evidence of reversing atherosclerosis. Another benefit of Delta tocotrienol is its ability to inhibit platelet aggregation which is a leading cause of heart attack. In addition, although taking a baby aspirin a day helps thin the blood, tocotrienols do the same thing without the risk of bleeding of the stomach.

Interestingly, the effect of delta tocotrienol vitamin E has been shown strongest when used independently of other vitamin E products. In a recent study, participants using tocotrienols without tocopherols recorded on an average 25% reduction of LDL cholesterol.

When choosing your supplements specifically to treat high cholesterol, it is recommended to verify that your supplement contains the delta tocotrienol form of vitamin E. When taking tocotrienols it is recommended that you should also take CoQ10.

(Reasons of using CoQ10 and Vitamin E together are explained below)

Recommended dosages vary, but experts suggest 100 milligrams of tocotrienols and 60 mg of CoQ10. As with any supplement, consult with your physician before taking.

12.   CoQ10

CoQ10 is a fat-soluble, vitamin-like compound found in all of your body's cells. You can get it from foods like broccoli, cabbage, ocean fish, meats, and nuts, but mostly your body makes it internally. But like a lot of other nutrients, the body slows down in making CoQ10 around age 20. CoQ10 is an energy booster. As an antioxidant, it helps prevent cellular damage. Supplementation has been suggested as a way to maintain the benefits of coenzyme.

CoQ10 travels along in the blood with LDL cholesterol working as an antioxidant by generating energy from oxygen. When vitamin E is used alone there is actually an increase in oxidation, so CoQ10 utilizes this energy and promotes cellular health, rather than allowing free radical damage. CoQ10 and tocotrienols work synergistically to nourish heart health.

Recommended dosages vary, but experts suggest 100 milligrams of tocotrienols and 60 mg of CoQ10. As with any supplement, consult with your physician before taking.

13.   Policosanol

Policosanol is a natural supplement derived from sugar cane wax and beeswax. In a number of studies over the past 10 years, it has proved effective at reducing cholesterol levels. The American Heart Journal is quoted as saying policosanol is "a very promising phytochemical alternative to classic lipid-lowering agents such as statins." In its study, policosanol was seen to lower total cholesterol by up to 21%, to lower LDL cholesterol by up to 29%, and to raise HDL cholesterol by up to 15%.

Participants in these most recent studies took policosanol in doses of 10-20 mg a day. But this supplement causes weight loss.

Note: Because policosanol can thin the blood as much as aspirin, if you are taking blood thinners, consult your primary care physician before taking policosanol. As with any supplement, consult with your physician before taking.

14. Folic Acid

Folic acid is a B vitamin. It is used in our bodies to make new cells. However, studies have shown that patients who suffer from high levels of cholesterol can significantly benefit from the antioxidant properties of the vitamin.

Research has shown that participants who supplemented their diets with folic acid for just four weeks were able to see an increased flexibility in their blood vessels and the ability of their blood vessels to dilate more easily. Both of these findings are extremely positive in showing the beneficial effects of folic acid in minimizing the damaging effects of high cholesterol.

Folic acid is naturally found in green leafy vegetables. Eating more green leafy vegetables is recommended.

15. Check your drinking water

Chlorine is being added to the drinking water since the late 80s to prevent waterborne disease. While the positive effects of chlorinating water seem obvious (as a disinfectant to keep us from getting sick), many experts have demonstrated that chlorine may actually do much more harm than good. For many years, it has been known that chlorine can have harmful side effects that relate to heart disease.

Chlorine leads to excess free radicals. Free radicals left unchecked lead to cell damage. Once the cells have been damaged, we see atherosclerosis, hardening of the arteries, and plaque formation—each of which can have potentially life-threatening impacts.

Invest in a water filtration system that not only removes chlorine, but also Trihalomethanes (THM) which includes cancer causing agents such as chloroforms, bromoforms, and carbontectachloride. Preferably use distilled water or water that has been treated by both reverse osmosis and carbon/charcoal treatments.

16. Carnitine (L=Carnitine)

Carnitine is a nutrient that helps the body convert fatty acids into energy. The body naturally produces carnitine in the liver and kidneys. It is observed that persons who took carnitine saw significant lowering of their total cholesterol and triglycerides, and an increase in their HDL (good) cholesterol levels. But avoid red meat with high saturated fat, particularly lamb, and dairy though they are the highest sources of carnitine. However, it can also be found in fish, asparagus, avocados, and peanut butter. In addition, carnitine is available as a supplement in a variety of forms, but only the form L-carnitine is recommended. Recommended dosages vary, but experts suggest 600 to 1,200 mg three times daily, or 750 mg twice daily.

As with any supplement, consult with your physician before taking.

17.   Pantethine

Pantethine is derived from pantothenic acid (vitamin B5and tries to maintain normal levels of cholesterol and triglycerides. It has been observed that Pantethine can significantly reduce serum triglyceride by up to 32%, total cholesterol by up to 19% and LDL cholesterol by up to 21%, while increasing HDL cholesterol up to 23%. There does not appear to be any side effects from Pantethine.

Recommended dosages vary, but experts suggest 300 mg three times a day.

Chapter 7

Prevention of Heart Attack

Heart disease remains the number one cause of death for both men and women in the United States.

Even surgical procedures like coronary artery bypass and angioplasty do not cure heart disease. It's important to look at your lifestyle to see if you're doing all you can to take care of your heart. Diet and exercise are always factors within your control. So is stress management.

And making sure your heart has a steady energy supply cannot be underestimated. The most fundamental process that fuels your heart is the release of energy when ATP breaks down in the cell. Anything you do to support that process will make your heart beat stronger and more efficiently. You can't take ATP in a pill, but you can give your cells what they need to make it happen.

ATP is a molecule that stores energy like a rechargeable battery. It is literally your cellular – and your life's – energy supply. But the thing about energy is that it is not a compound. It's a force. It happens as a result of a chemical reaction.

When the ATP molecule is broken down, it releases its energy and turns into adenosine diphosphate (ADP). All that means is that the molecule went from having three phosphates to two. It is the breaking off of the third phosphate that releases the energy force.

Fortunately, the body can recycle ADP back into ATP by adding that third phosphate back. It does this by rebuilding the molecule with nutrients and oxygen delivered by the blood stream. It's a constant process that needs to stay in balance. If production and recycling of ATP slows down, the energy level of the cell drops, much like a battery losing its charge.

Since energy is a force, you can't put it in a pill or a drink. You have to supply the raw materials the body needs to make and re-charge ATP. ATP is not a vitamin or a mineral you can take with breakfast. It's constantly made and recycled in all your cells.

Dr. Sinatra discovered how to enhance and restore the ATP energy process.

So what are the raw materials that help form ATP in the cells? Dr. Sinatra calls them the "awesome foursome," and they each play a vital role in providing cellular energy. They are:

· Coenzyme Q10

· L-carnitine

· D-ribose

· Magnesium

The mitochondria require a good supply of each one of these compounds to generate ATP. Let's take a closer look at how each one works.

CoQ10

CoQ10 is a fat-soluble, vitamin-like compound found in all of your body's cells. You can get it from foods like broccoli, cabbage, ocean fish, meats, and nuts, but mostly your body makes it internally. But like a lot of other nutrients, the body slows down in making CoQ10 around age twenty. CoQ10 is an energy booster. It is what provides the spark in the mitochondria that sets off the release of energy by ATP. And since the heart is the pump that keeps the body going, it has a tremendous need for CoQ10 to circulate the blood. In fact, tissue levels of CoQ10 are up to ten times higher in a healthy heart than any other organ of the body.

People with congestive heart failure (CHF) are often low in CoQ10. CHF occurs when the heart doesn't pump the blood very well. This causes blood to pool in parts of the body like the lungs and the legs. Studies have shown that CoQ10 can reduce leg swelling and reduce fluid in the lungs by energizing the heart to pump stronger.

One study using CoQ10 for congestive heart failure followed 2,664 patients. After taking 100 mg of CoQ10 daily for three months, fluid retention was reduced by79%. Lung congestion was reduced by 78%, heart palpitations were reduced by 75% and shortness of breath was reduced by 53%.

CoQ10 not only improves energy production in cells, it inhibits blood clot formation. People who take daily CoQ10 supplements within three days of a heart attack are less likely to have chest pain or another heart attack. They are also less likely to die of heart disease than those who do not get the supplement.

CoQ10 is also a powerful antioxidant. Taking CoQ10 prior to heart surgery reduces damage caused by free radicals. It strengthens the heart and helps regulate the heart beat during recovery.

And a good oxygen supply allows the heart to work more efficiently.

Medications that deplete CoQ10 in the body include statin drugs (used to lower cholesterol) and beta blockers. Taking supplements can correct the deficiency and can also decrease the muscle pain often caused by statin treatment.

Production of CoQ10 in the body really drops after age 80, which correlates with a higher incidence of congestive heart failure. The older heart is very vulnerable to stress and lack of oxygen, but one study showed that CoQ10 could increase the workload an older heart can sustain by 28%.

D-Ribose - Sweetness in Action

D-ribose is a kind of sugar produced by the body. It is found in every cell and is often used as a medicine because it boosts muscle energy. It also helps prevents cramping, pain and stiffness after exercise.

Unlike the other compounds of the "awesome foursome," D-ribose is a structural component needed to make the ATP reactions happen. But D-ribose is an actual ingredient. That means it is a building block that helps rebuild energy within the cell.

Ribose is found naturally in the body, but it cannot be stored in cells. Cells actually have to make ribose every time it is needed. And because it is a sugar, it is metabolized quickly. About 97% of supplemental ribose will be absorbed into the blood within 30 to 120 minutes. From there, it is easily transferred to tissue for energy. Because of this fast processing, ribose is quick fuel for the heart.

Ischemia (lack of oxygen) due to heart disease can cause a loss of 50% of the ATP energy pool in heart cells. Even when blood flow and oxygen are restored to a damaged heart, it can take up to ten days for the heart to rebuild its basic cellular energy. But when ribose is supplemented, the same process of energy recovery can happen in just one to two days.

. It also helps prevents cramping, pain and stiffness after exercise.

Unlike the other compounds of the "awesome foursome," D-ribose is a structural component of ATP. The other three compounds are "precursors" – elements.

L-carnitine - Turning Fat into Fuel

L-carnitine is a vitamin-type nutrient you can get from foods like red meat and dairy products. It is also produced naturally by the body, although that production tends to decrease with age.

L-carnitine helps the body produce energy by transporting fatty acids into the mitochondria to be burned for fuel. For the heart to keep beating 60 to 100 times every minute of every day, it needs a constant supply of fuel, so this energy transport is critical.

On the way back out of the cell, L-carnitine removes toxic by-products that interfere with energy production. It's like a bus that carries vital compounds into and out of the cell. It's a critical process since, for these compounds, it's the only way in or out. L-carnitine is also a vasodilator that helps keep blood vessels open. With better blood flow, oxygen gets delivered to the heart and all other parts of the body.

160 patients hospitalized with a heart attack were divided into two groups. 80 received 4 g of L-carnitine a day for 12 months. 80 received a placebo. This was in addition to standard treatment. All subjects had improvements in blood pressure, cholesterol and heart rhythm. However, the mortality rate in the L-carnitine group was 1.2% compared to 12.5% in the placebo group.

Because of the way L-carnitine improves cellular energy production, athletes often use it to enhance stamina and endurance. The added benefit is that L-carnitine also helps clear excess lactic acid from the body. This aids in recovery since lactic acid contributes to muscle pain and fatigue. Reducing lactic acid levels can relieve fatigue in heart patients as well.

Magnesium - the Rescue Mineral

Magnesium is the fourth most abundant mineral in your body. It is most concentrated in the mitochondria and plays a vital role in ATP production. It also helps keep blood vessels open by relaxing the artery walls.

Because of the relaxation effect, magnesium can help lower blood pressure. A study where participants took 300mg of magnesium a day for three months confirmed this. The systolic/diastolic pressure in those who took the magnesium fell 17.1/6.7 mmHg compared to 3.4/0.8 in the placebo group.[16]

Adequate intake of magnesium also lowers risk of sudden cardiac death. Researchers at Brigham and Women's Hospital of Harvard Medical School reviewed 26 years of data from The Nurses' Health Study. They found that those with the highest blood levels of magnesium had a 37% lower incidence of sudden cardiac death.

A great majority of people are deficient in magnesium regardless of dietary intake. If your diet doesn't include a lot of green leafy vegetables and fresh fruit, then you may be low in magnesium. A good baseline is to supplement with 400 mg per day. Try magnesium citrate since it is very inexpensive and is easily absorbed in the body.

Magnesium is found in green vegetables like spinach and whole grains, but most people don't get enough magnesium from food. Excess caffeine and alcohol washes magnesium out of the body, as do diuretics. People with congestive heart failure are often deficient in magnesium due to using diuretics to control fluid retention. This can lead to irregular heartbeat unless magnesium is replenished

Quick Guide for Using the Four Pillars of Heart Health...

General Protocol:

CoQ10:	90-150	mg	per	day
L-carnitine:	250-750	mg	per	day
D-ribose:	5	grams	per	day

Magnesium: 400 mg per day

High Blood Pressure:

CoQ10:	180-360	mg	per	day
L-carnitine:	500-1000	mg	per	day

D-ribose: 5-10 grams per day

Magnesium:	400-800	mg	per	day

Diagnosed Heart Disease:

CoQ10:	180-360	mg	per	day
L-carnitine:	1000-2000	mg	per	day
D-ribose:	7-10	grams	per	day

Magnesium: 400-800 mg per day

Note: you should work with your personal physician if you have any sort of heart disease and take medication for it. Generally, nutritional supplements are safe taken in appropriate doses, but they may have an interaction with some medications.

A Steady Energy Supply

1 + 1 + 1 + 1 = A whole lot more than four!

The four pillars of heart health – CoQ10, L-carnitine, D-ribose, and magnesium – are vital elements in the production of ATP (the source of energy) in every cell. They are particularly important in fueling the heart. So it's not surprising to find that people with heart problems are deficient in these nutrients.

But if each of these nutrients is a powerhouse on its own, it's amazing what happens when they all work together. They can literally refuel and recharge an energy-starved heart. None of the nutrients work alone. Each one depends on some function of another one to create a process that releases energy. It takes a constant supply of energy for the heart to pump. Energy is life.

Dr. James Roberts credits the four nutrients with keeping his patients out of the hospital. At one time, Dr. Roberts felt that nutritional medicine was "unproven." But after observing improvements in a friend who used CoQ10, he began to give it to his own patients. In combination with L-carnitine, his patients began showing remarkable improvements and he got fewer calls in the middle of the night.

Eventually Dr. Roberts added D-ribose to his patients' treatment regimens and saw even more improvement. In fact, he went from being the number one cardiology emergency room admitter in his primary hospital, to rarely even having a patient in the hospital at all! His heart failure readmission rate is almost zero and he seldom has to get out of bed in the middle of the night to see a sick patient.

Dr. Sinatra comments that he doesn't know how he ever practiced cardiovascular medicine without these four vital nutrients. They make such a difference in the quality of life for his patients that he would feel like he was withholding vital information if he didn't use nutritional therapies.

CHAPTER 8
Conclusion

Though Cholesterol is required for health of the body, it must be kept in healthy range. Increase of LDL beyond this range can create Heart problem depending on other factors like age, gender, life style, weight, and genetics. It is important that we must keep LDL and VLDL strictly under control and increase HDL to prevent any heart problem. We should get regular blood tested and eat healthy food and avoid saturated fats and trans-fat. We should quit smoking and eat vegetables and fruits as far as possible and exercise regularly. Pranayam (breathing exercises) especially alternative breathing (known as Lome Prolome) can help in control of Cholesterol.

By adopting healthy life, we can not only prevent but also cure heart problems and increase our life span.

Further after certain age we should include required supplements for remaining healthy and prevention of heart problem.

About author

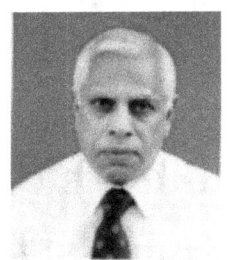

V.K.Grover has about 20 years' experience in Alternative Treatments and have cured many persons through Natural treatment and Reiki.

He is qualified Reiki Master and Pranic Healer.

He has authored 3 other books in Kindle and paper back. Books are

1. **Manage High Blood Pressure naturally and stop taking medicines.**
2. **Self-Examination-Diagnose your Health by Self-observation.**
3. **How to heal and prevent diseases.**

These books help in natural diagnosis and cure.

He regularly publishes blogs and research reports on his site www.freelycure.com

www.ingramcontent.com/pod-product-compliance
Lightning Source LLC
Chambersburg PA
CBHW071838200526
45169CB00020B/1832